Gutsy Sex for Men
Sex & Intimacy in 4 Realms

This 'Gutsy Sex' Guide is designed to help men discover the unique sexual needs in their marriages and to teach them to *'cherishingly hold female hearts'* with clean hands.

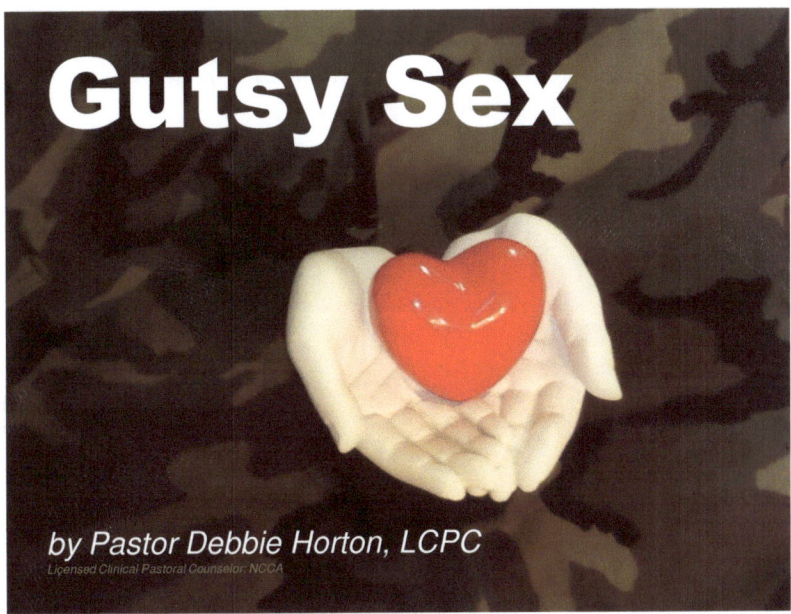

Some of the material in this LifeCare Guide is sexually explicit. It comes from the Bible, scientific research and human experiences. As you read the material ask the Holy Spirit to teach you what is useful and acceptable for you and your spouse. Remember that your goal is always to love and please God in all you do.

DEDICATION

LifeCare Guides are dedicated to helping people live fulfilling and satisfying lives that honor God. As you read these guides may you find peace and freedom to function in life per your unique God-design.

With gratitude and humility these guides are written from life experiences, education, research, training and the influence of those who have loved me, as well as those who have not been able to love me.

To purchase an Assessment Package and other LifeCare Guides written by the LifeCare team and Pastor Debbie Horton, LCPC go to:

www.lifecarecounselors.com and www.amazon.com

CONTENTS

For most women, sexual interest starts when she feels her heart being held in a cherishing manner by the clean hands of her husband.

BIBLE VERSES ABOUT SEX

"...The body is not meant for sexual immorality, but for the Lord, and the Lord for the body...Do you not know that your bodies are members of Christ himself? Shall I then take the members of Christ and unite them with a prostitute? Never! Do you not know that he who unites himself with a prostitute is one with her in body? For it is said 'the two will become one flesh' ..." [I Corinthians 6:13-16]

"The husband should fulfill his marital duty to his wife, and likewise the wife to her husband. The wife's body does not belong to her alone but also to her husband. In the same way, the husband's body does not belong to him alone but also to his wife. Do not deprive each other except by mutual consent and for a time, so that you may devote yourselves to prayer. Then come together again so that Satan will not tempt you because of your lack of self-control." [I Corinthians 7:3-5]

"But if they cannot control themselves, they should marry, for it is better to marry than to burn with passion." [I Corinthians 7:9]
"For a man's ways are in full view of the Lord, and he examines all his paths. The evil deeds of a wicked man ensnare him; the cords of his sin hold him fast. He will die for lack of discipline, led astray by his own great folly." [Proverbs 5:15-23]

"Like an apple tree among the trees of the forest is my lover among the young men. I delight to sit in his shade and his fruit is sweet to my taste. He has taken me to the banquet hall, and his banner over me is love. Strengthen me with raisins, refresh me with apples, for I am faint with love. His left arm is under my head, and his right arm embraces me. Daughters of Jerusalem, I charge you by the gazelles and by the does of the field: Do not arouse or awaken love until it so desires."   [Song of Songs 2:3-7]

"How beautiful you are, my darling! Oh, how beautiful! Your eyes behind your veil are doves. Your hair is like a flock of goats descending from Mount Gilead. Your teeth are like a flock of sheep just shorn, coming up from the washing.

Each has its twin; not one of them is alone. Your lips are like a scarlet ribbon; your mouth is lovely. Your temples behind your veil are like the halves of a pomegranate. Your neck is like a tower of David. built with elegance; on it hang a thousand shields, all of them shields of warriors. Your two breasts are like two fawns, like twin fawns of a gazelle that browse among the lilies. Until the day breaks and the shadows flee, I will go to the mountain of myrrh and to the hill of incense. All beautiful you are my darling; there is no flaw in you." [Song of Songs 4:1-7]

"My lover is radiant and ruddy, outstanding among ten thousand. His head is purest gold; his hair is wavy and black as a raven. His eyes are like doves by the water streams, washed in milk, mounted like jewels. His cheeks are like beds of spice yielding perfume. His lips are like lilies dripping with myrrh. His arms are rods of gold set with chrysolite. His body is like polished ivory decorated with sapphires. His legs are pillars of marble set on bases of pure gold. His appearance is like Lebanon, choice as its cedars. His mouth is sweetness itself; he is altogether lovely. This is my lover, this my friend..." [Song of Songs 5:10-16]

"You are beautiful, my darling, as Tirzah, lovely as Jerusalem, majestic as troops with banners. Turn your eyes from me; they overwhelm me. Your hair is like a flock of goats descending from Gilead. Your teeth are like a flock of sheep coming up from the washing. Each has its twin, not one of them is alone. Your temples behind your veil are like the halves of a pomegranate. Sixty queens there may be, and eighty concubines, and virgins beyond number; but my dove, my perfect one, is unique, the only daughter of her mother, the favorite of the one who bore her. The maidens saw her and called her blessed; the queens and concubines praised her." [Song of Songs 6:4-9]

"Your stature is like that of the palm, and your breasts like clusters of fruit. I said, "I will climb the palm tree; I will take hold of its fruit." May your breasts be like the clusters of the vine, the fragrance of your breath like apples, and your mouth like the best wine. May the wine go straight to my lover, flowing gently over lips and teeth. I belong to my lover, and his desire is for me." [Song of Songs 7:7-10]

"I am a wall and my breasts are like towers. Thus I have become in his eyes like one bringing contentment." [Song of Songs 8:10]

"You have heard that it was said, 'You shall not commit adultery.' But I say to you that everyone who looks at a woman with lustful intent has already committed adultery with her in his heart. If your right eye causes you to sin, tear it out and throw it away. For it is better that you lose one of your members than that your whole body be thrown into hell. And if your right hand causes you to sin, cut it off and throw it away. For it is better that you lose one of your members than that your whole body go into hell. [*Matthew 5:27-30*]

For this reason God gave them up to dishonorable passions. For their women exchanged natural relations for those that are contrary to nature; and the men likewise gave up natural relations with women and were consumed with passion for one another, men committing shameless acts with men and receiving in themselves the due penalty for their error. [*Romans 1:26-27*]

Or do you not know that the unrighteous will not inherit the kingdom of God? Do not be deceived: neither the sexually immoral, nor idolaters, nor adulterers, nor men who practice homosexuality, nor thieves, nor the greedy, nor drunkards, nor revilers, nor swindlers will inherit the kingdom of God. And such were some of you. But you were washed, you were sanctified, you were justified in the name of the Lord Jesus Christ and by the Spirit of our God.

"All things are lawful for me," but not all things are helpful. "All things are lawful for me," but I will not be enslaved by anything. "Food is meant for the stomach and the stomach for food"—and God will destroy both one and the other. The body is not meant for sexual immorality, but for the Lord, and the Lord for the body. And God raised the Lord and will also raise us up by his power. Do you not know that your bodies are members of Christ? Shall I then take the members of Christ and make them members of a prostitute? Never! Or do you not know that he who is joined to a prostitute becomes one body with her?

For, as it is written, "The two will become one flesh." But he who is joined to the Lord becomes one spirit with him. Flee from sexual immorality. Every other sin a person commits is outside the body, but the sexually immoral person sins against his own body. Or do you not know that your body is a temple of the Holy Spirit within you, whom you have from God? You are not your own, for you were bought with a price. So glorify God in your body. [*1 Corinthians 6:9-20*]

But I say, walk by the Spirit, and you will not gratify the desires of the flesh. For the desires of the flesh are against the Spirit, and the desires of the Spirit are against the flesh, for these are opposed to each other, to keep you from doing the things you want to do. But if you are led by the Spirit, you are not under the law. Now the works of the flesh are evident: sexual immorality, impurity, sensuality, idolatry, sorcery, enmity, strife, jealousy, fits of anger, rivalries, dissensions, divisions, envy, drunkenness, orgies, and things like these. I warn you, as I warned you before, that those who do such things will not inherit the kingdom of God. [Galatians 5:16-21]

They have become callous and have given themselves up to sensuality, greedy to practice every kind of impurity. But that is not the way you learned Christ!— assuming that you have heard about him and were taught in him, as the truth is in Jesus, to put off your old self, which belongs to your former manner of life and is corrupt through deceitful desires, and to be renewed in the spirit of your minds, and to put on the new self, created after the likeness of God in true righteousness and holiness. [Ephesians 4:19-24]

But sexual immorality and all impurity or covetousness must not even be named among you, as is proper among saints. Let there be no filthiness nor foolish talk nor crude joking, which are out of place, but instead let there be thanksgiving. For you may be sure of this, that everyone who is sexually immoral or impure, or who is covetous (that is, an idolater), has no inheritance in the kingdom of Christ and God. [*Ephesians 5:3-5*]

For this is the will of God, your sanctification: that you abstain from sexual immorality; that each one of you know how to control his own body in holiness and honor, not in the passion of lust like the Gentiles who do not know God; that no one transgress and wrong his brother in this matter, because the Lord is an avenger in all these things, as we told you beforehand and solemnly warned you. For God has not called us for impurity, but in holiness. Therefore whoever disregards this, disregards not man but God, who gives his Holy Spirit to you.
[*1 Thessalonians 4:3-8*]

Let marriage be held in honor among all, and let the marriage bed be undefiled, for God will judge the sexually immoral and adulterous.
[*Hebrews 13:4*]

But as for the cowardly, the faithless, the detestable, as for murderers, the sexually immoral, sorcerers, idolaters, and all liars, their portion will be in the lake that burns with fire and sulfur, which is the second death." [*Revelation 21:8*]

INTIMACY IN FOUR REALMS
HELPS CREATE 'GUTSY SEX'

Jesus said to Love in all Four Realms: Spiritual, Emotional, Mental & Physical (Mark 12:30-31). 'Gutsy Sex' is Intimacy in Four Realms with all Six Senses Engaged. This is "Gutsy" because it requires risking open vulnerability.

1ST Spiritual Relationship Wholeness & Intimacy **(heart)**
Focus on Faith Intimacy: Connect to God & each other through prayer, communion, spiritual sharing, studying the Bible together
(Recommended Reading: The Bible, Wired for Intimacy, Pure Desire)

2ND Emotional Relationship Wholeness & Intimacy **(soul)**
Focus on Feeling Intimacy: Communicate at least 30 min. a day minimum, share feelings openly with each other, explore feelings together, honor all feelings
(Recommended Reading: Journey to the Other Side of Life)

3RD Mental Relationship Wholeness & Intimacy **(mind)**
Focus on Thought Intimacy: Discuss your views & opinions together, explore & understand your personal missions and goals in life, talk about interests
(Recommended Reading: Discovering the Mind of a Woman)

4TH Physical Relationship Wholeness & Intimacy **(strength)**
Focus on Action Intimacy: Spend time & energy together, physically touch each other, sit next to each other, hold hands, hug, snuggle, go on walks, date, travel, take a bath together, massage each other, have sexual intercourse
(Recommended Reading: Intended for Pleasure)

'Gutsy Sex' takes two WHOLE people living in connection and unity as they love one another in all four realms. God said the two shall become one flesh (Matt 19:5). It takes two WHOLE people for 'GUTSY SEX'. Do whatever you can to get help to improve your relationship if you are not experiencing intimacy in all 4 realms. There is no shame in asking for help. It is okay to need one another and seek assistance.

ENGAGEMENT OF THE SIX SENSES

Begin by creating your own "Bedside Essentials" to help you engage all six senses during sexual intimacy with your spouse. Purchase or imagine six different colored gift bags. You will fill each one with the essentials (tools) to assist you in being aware of the need to engage all six senses. Listed here are some of the examples to help you design your own 'Gutsy Sex' "Bedside Essentials".

1st sense is Intuitive - Red Bag to represent the Intuitive Sense
These can help you with developing healthy connection in all 4 Realms and create a sense of safety, belonging and unity (Bible & Books for spiritual growth, Communion & Anointing Oil for Prayer together, Love Coupons, Locked Doors to prevent interruptions, Calendar to schedule time together, etc.)

2nd sense is Smell — Pink Bag to represent the sense of smell
Cleanliness and pleasant odors (lotions, cologne, room spray, candles, etc.)

3rd sense is Visual — Purple Bag to represent the visual sense
Visually pleasing atmosphere (dimmer switch, colored lights, flowers, lingerie, dress-up surprises, press-on tattoos, beads, bubbles, blindfold, fan dance, nude modeling for each other, etc.)

4th sense is Auditory — Silver Bag to represent auditory sense
Soothing & Sensual Sounds (no noisy kids, mood music, waterfall sounds, pouring a beverage and clicking the glasses, words of love, read a love note or poetry, sexual sounds of satisfaction, etc.)

5th sense is Taste — Green Bag to represent the sense of taste
Entice the Taste Buds: (breath mints, chocolates, flavored lip gloss & lotions, favorite beverage, whip crème, chocolate, cherries, etc.)

6th sense is Touch — Gold Bag to represent the sense of touch
Stimulating Touch: (room temperature, clean comfy bed, kiss, cuddle, massage, fingernails, extra pillows, feathers, games, sex toys, vibrators, chux and wipes for cleanup, etc.)

WHAT'S the DIFFERENCE?
How to Grow in Relationship Wholeness and Intimacy

The need to understand ourselves and one another is vital to growing in unity. Understanding each other can help us respond correctly. When we respond instead of react, we can begin to flow in unity. Group dynamics affect people's ability to relate to one another in a particular group. Understanding yourself and the uniqueness of others empowers effective daily living.

Consider the following areas where we differ from each other. Use this list of questions to gain an understanding of your behaviors and the behaviors of others. Depending on the answers to these questions, each person responds differently to the same situation or circumstance. When four different people witness an automobile accident, the police often get four very different stories about what really happened. The same is true with our relationships with one another. We just don't always see things from the same point of view. And that's Okay!

1   What are your unique spiritual needs? (gifts, calling, ministry)
2   What are your unique needs (mental, emotional, spiritual, skills, etc.
3   What is your birth order? (birth order affects our response)
4   What are your ethnic & social backgrounds? (tradition, world view, etc.)
5   What was your childhood like? (family of origin affects us)
6   What are your educational background, training, and experience?
7   Do you know your purpose in life?
8   What are some of your personal triumphs and tragedies?
9   What is your marital and relationship status? (repeated conflicts, etc.)
10 What is your occupation or career?
11 What are your interests and hobbies?
12 What's your church background? (pleasant, painful, denominations, etc.)
13 What is your financial status? (comfortable, stressed)
14 How is your physical condition? (age, diet, habits, health, etc.)
15 How is your mental state? (stressed, low morale, intellectually tired)
16 How is your emotional state? (happy, hurting, loneliness, depressed)
17 How is your spiritual growth? (character qualities, forgiveness, fruits)
18 How is your self-image? (physical, emotional, mental, and spiritual)
19 What are your desires, goals, and visions?
20 What are your greatest fears, frustrations and concerns?

Take time to learn about yourself and others. Learn to understand differences and how to respond in healthy ways.

The difficulty in obtaining unity is often due to a lack of understanding yourself and other people. Understanding one another helps us come into "oneness" and set goals and see plans and visions that will fulfill God's purposes. All of us naturally desire wholeness and health but often lack the skills and tools to help us discover and understand how to reach them. When we learn to Experience and Extend Love we begin to move out of a dysfunctional mentality into a **L**.ife **O**.ccupation **V**.alued **E**.ternally through serving and loving ourselves, others and God. (Mark 12:30-31)

As fellow human beings, we should not focus on our differences as obstacles or irritations, but as unique and precious aspects of God's creation. Differences are an opportunity to see more of God and to Experience and Extend Love in a variety of ways. Once we understand other people's differences, responses and reactions, it is much easier to find ways to help them meet their own needs without sacrificing our needs. Remember that learning about your uniqueness and responses, as well as understanding others, will help to empower effective daily living where you Experience and Extend Love regularly.

There are other LifeCare Guides that can help you discover your personal unique needs and provide you with numerous tools to assist in developing more life empowerment skills. For information on purchasing other LifeCare Guides written by Pastor Debbie Horton, LCPC go to: www.lifecarecounselors.com and www.amazon.com

SEXUAL TENDENCIES OF UNIQUE TEMPERAMENTS

Just like people, marriages do not have the same DNA. So how could sex be the same in every marriage? Our unique temperament affects our sexual tendencies, as you will understand as you read these varied traits.

Supine Affection Strengths: the ability to respond to love and to open up emotionally when they feel emotionally 'safe.' If treated properly, they are capable of absolute and total commitment to deep personal relationships.

Supine Affection Weaknesses: the inability to initiate love and affection. They require constant reassurance that they are loved, needed and appreciated.

Sanguine Affection Strengths: Able to express and receive large amounts of love and affection. They are warm and easy to get to know and emotionally open.

Sanguine Affection Weaknesses: Easily devastated if not constantly reassured they are loved and appreciated. Very demanding of other people for love and affection, plagued with feeling of jealousy when the love and attention they feel belongs exclusively to them is given to others.

Melancholy Affection Strengths: very faithful, loyal friends and self-sacrificing. Their feelings run deep and tender (even though they lack the ability to express these feelings). They easily empathize with others and have an ability to make very deep commitments.

Melancholy Affection Weaknesses: They dissect the past, worry about being more loveable, critical of others, angry, cruel, vengeful, emotional, rarely tell people how they feel, have a low self-image and are sensitive to rejection from deep relationships. The loss of a deep relationship (even by death) is devastating to them. They are not romantically inclined and this causes marital problems.

Choleric Affection Strengths: being open, optimistic, outgoing, express a great deal of love and affection, and approach only select people for deep relationships.

Choleric Affection Weaknesses: extremely self-centered (although they do not appear this way), indirect behavior, reject people, reject the love and affections of people (they will accept love and affection only according to their terms), are usually cruel to those who reject their manipulation for love and affection.

Phlegmatic Affection Strengths: well balanced, easygoing, non-demanding, calm and realistic in demands for love and affection.

Phlegmatic Affection Weaknesses: unwillingness to become involved in deep relationships, tendency to be an observer only, rarely self-sacrificing, unemotional and inexpressive. Verbal defenses are used to protect low energy supply with regard to physical and sexual involvement.

If you don't know your unique temperament and emotional needs, you can order an online assessment at our website: www.lifecarecounselors.com

FEELINGS ABOUT SEX

Before, during and after sex what emotions do you experience? This chart is a small sampling of some possible feelings. Take a few minutes to explore how you feel about sex. Your emotions help reveal your needs, thoughts and beliefs regarding sexuality. Feelings can help you become more aware of yourself and your needs. Once you identify your emotions it can help you work on changing thoughts and beliefs to find healthy ways to get your needs met. In some cases, you may need a counselor to assist with this journey.

Happiness	Fear	Anger	Guilt
Good	Uneasy	Irritated	At Fault
Happy	Shy	Annoyed	Wrong
Glad	Timid	Agitated	Sorry
On Track	Insecure	Frustrated	Regretful
Safe	Cautious	Grouchy	Ashamed
Accepted	Apprehensive	Rejecting	Remorseful
Noticed	Worried	Mad	Awful
Hopeful	Bashful	Ticked Off	Bad
Cared for	Inhibited	Fed Up	Self-Disgust
Connected	Reluctant	Furious	Soul Searching
Trusting	Risky	Resentful	Self-Hate
Lovable	Anxious	Get Back	Judged
Loving	Afraid	Get Even	Condemned
Valued	Coward	Provoked	Self-Punishing
Important	Guarded	Pushed	Self-Destructive
Capable	Dreading	Livid	To Blame
Competent	Panicky	Hostile	Guilty
Strong	Terrified	Violent	In Error
Confident	Horrified	Aggravated	Shamed
Intelligent	Boxed in	Grumpy	Appalling
Recognized	Uptight	Upset	Foul
Appreciated	Restless	Cranky	Ghastly
Celebrated	Nervous	Cynical	Unpleasant
Honored	Overwhelmed	Burnt Up	Dirty
Committed	Panic Stricken	Indignant	Ruined
Self Directed	Hysterical	Infuriated	Contaminated
Powerful	Petrified	Rage	Polluted
Free	Intimidated	Resentment	Impure

INTIMACY (In – To – Me- See)

"In-To-Me-See" in my Spiritual Realm
"In-To-Me-See" in my Emotional Realm
"In-To-Me-See" in my Mental Realm
"In-To-Me-See" in my Physical Realm

True *intimacy* means you know, understand and accept yourself and other people in all four realms of life. True *intimacy* means you are connected and fully present in the moment with yourself and the other. This includes your relationship with God. It is living honesty, in the moment, one day at a time, by loving and 'being' your Authentic Self.

The single biggest problem with most relationships is that there are too many people involved for True *intimacy* to occur. For instance: A romantic relationship is supposed to be two people in partnership sharing who they are, sharing their hearts, minds, bodies, and souls with each other. Anyone who has **not** done their own emotional healing is bringing an overabundance of people into any relationship they get involved in. Some of these people can include: parents, siblings, relatives; ministers, teachers, the junior high school bully; everyone that they have ever had a romantic relationship with; the Prince and Princess of fairy tales, the lyrics of songs, and the characters from books and movies. Just to think of how many "ghosts" are in the room, when two 'unaware' people are interacting, is mind boggling.

Anyone who is unconscious (unaware) of how the people and events of their past have shaped who they are today, is incapable of being present in the now and having a healthy relationship with themselves and with others. When we are reacting unconsciously to the emotional wounds and old tapes from our childhoods, we are being emotionally dishonest in the moment - we are mostly reacting to how we felt in a similar dynamic in the past, not clearly responding to what is happening in the present.

The single most important component in a healthy relationship is the ability to communicate in healthy ways. We cannot communicate clearly and functionally when we are reacting because we are not being emotionally honest with ourselves. Any person who reacts defensively has not been working on healing their own emotional wounds.

Our goal with each other should be to help one another become conscious (aware) of our unique needs, beliefs and process of relating. A supportive environment will allow the necessary healing and recovery to develop and grow. Focusing on learning good communication tools and new relationship skills facilitates healthy, satisfying relationships with God, with themselves and with others.

Enjoying "In-To-Me-See" in our relationships is Experiencing and Extending Love. This makes God known and visible and is the greatest calling.

True *intimacy* is a **L**.ife **O**.ccupation **V**.alued **E**.ternally

LIMBIC RESONANCE & REVISION

The limbic portion of the brain governs feelings. If our limbic patterning is off when it comes to loving, we can suffer endless trouble and repeated errors in relationships. The qualities of character, personality and behavior are etched into our psyche early and indelibly. We are created by God to need limbic resonance with others, that loving connection in relationships that we reach for time and time again throughout our lives.

The need for a loving connection whispers to us from beneath our veil of consciousness. We are unconsciously driven to search for ways to Experience and Extend Love; with God, with others and with our selves.

Sadly, some people grew up in homes, families, communities, and even churches, where the limbic blueprints placed in their brains early in life where not loving. This now leads them subconsciously to relationships where the other is often abusive, belittling, judgmental, critical and rejecting. There is hope. **Limbic Revision**, permitting wiser choices in relationships, is possible. Therapy can help. The particular type of therapy is less important than the therapist's making a good limbic imprint on the patient and changing the patient's taste in relationships.

Unfortunately, limbic revision takes time and hard work to create new 'wiring'. As brains age, they lose their plasticity. It is important that each of us helps every child in our lives experience healthy, loving limbic resonance, before they are adults.

As adults, to see real limbic revision often means long-term treatment with a trained therapist who understands the healing power of a loving connection, and has the skills to build that kind of relationship. God can heal in an instant, but He often uses people to bring the healing.

Loving is synchronous attunement and modulation. As Christians our main goal needs to be to provide loving, supportive connections with each person we encounter. Even though rewiring a broken limbic system isn't simple, it is possible. We can learn 'tangible' ways to share the 'love of Christ' with others through the ministry of relationships.

Healing will come in time as the person builds trust in the healing relationship. The real joy and reward is in seeing people set free to love others. If we, the Church, can begin to love each other with the kind of attunement and loving connection that Christ modeled, the world will know Him; through our love for one another. (John 17)

We spend a lot of our time learning about the environment around us, so that we can improve our quality of life by creating a better fit with it. Unfortunately, however, often we don't spend as much time to get to know ourselves, taking our behaviors, feelings and body responses for granted, staying on the surface, rather than exploring the depths of our being. In so doing, we risk living a very superficial life, with little understanding and thus little ability to change those behaviors that are less than optimal and yet we keep repeating over and over again, because we don't have enough self-awareness to create healthier choices for ourselves.

Getting acquainted with who we are, on the other hand, allows us to maintain an ongoing connection with our thoughts, feelings, motivations, conflicts and desires. It helps us make informed decisions about what is good, appropriate and healthy for us, by explaining to us where our attractions, repulsions, impulses and wishes, as well as fears come from. It provides us with room to reflect on our experiences; it helps us put things in perspective, and be able to better anticipate and prepare for the future.

It also gives us information about how to respond to different challenges; how we are affected by certain experiences, who and what we resonate with, and who and what we find alien to us. And, knowing ourselves enriches not only us but our intimate relationships as well, because by raising our awareness and sensitivity, it provides us with better ways of empathizing, communicating and sharing with our intimate relationships.

By the time we are adults, most of our emotional triggers are ones we have learned through our life experience. Emotions come on much more quickly than awareness does. Emotions direct us quickly, particularly in danger. Our fear and anger responses can happen in milliseconds, long before we are aware of them. Our awareness takes time to catch up.

We become aware that we are angry when we find our inner landscape already stormy with anger, rather than see it coming from a distance and decide to feel it.

We are always signaling our emotions with our facial expressions and bodily postures. People's emotions flicker quickly across their faces. When they try to conceal them, an honest display flickers for an instant and we can learn to read that.

People feel emotions at different levels of intensity. We also vary in how long an emotion will grip us. Some people are quicker to anger than others, and some naturally hold onto it for much longer than others.

Researchers say we have seven basic emotions: anger, disgust, sadness, contempt, happiness, fear and surprise. Some of them, particularly happiness, have many variations.

Emotional memories are stored in the limbic system, which combines them with an innate trigger to make an assessment of a situation automatically and below our threshold of awareness. Say we see a man on the street coming towards us and acting aggressive.

The limbic system will assess the threat. If it decides there is danger, it alerts the stress hormone system. It also sends a message to the neocortex, so that we think, "This guy's dangerous," and start to plan a response. Further, it alerts the part of the brain that controls breathing and blood flow, to prepare our fight, flight or freeze stress response.

The limbic system has a memory completely separate from the memory in the neocortex. In our neocortex we learn multiplication tables and the names of streets and people. The limbic system has an emotional filing system, indexing memories by their value for future experience. While the neocortex forgets, the **limbic system does not forget**.

The limbic system keeps increasing the data on which we depend. We forget telephone numbers stored in the neocortex. We don't forget what the limbic system knows—that we love our parents and our children. This capacity of the limbic system to keep building files may be why we lose data but gain wisdom as we age.

We are not aware of the limbic system as it collates its emotional memories and reaches conclusions. Researchers now think that **intuition emerges from this limbic process**. As our limbic mind reaches a conclusion, we feel pressure gather in our solar plexus. This nicely explains the colloquial notion that an intuition is a "gut feeling".

Emotions jump brains in a way that ideas do not. Our limbic systems are sensitive antennas to the emotions of other people. We can often feel emotional hostility at a distance. On the opposite pole, people say they can 'feel love' fill the room when loving people are present.

This ability to feel the feelings of others and to project our own is called Limbic Resonance.

It has particular importance for babies. When babies are born, their brains are only partly grown. A baby's limbic system must resonate with the mothers for its brain to grow properly. In extreme situations where there is little contact, the brain grows only partially, and will never be healthy. The resonance between the mother's and baby's limbic systems begins in the womb and continues to deepen after birth. Every baby imprints on its mother like it will on no one else. Its limbic system is hungry for resonance.

Beyond guaranteeing physical brain growth, the baby's brain learns its basic emotional expression by tuning to the mother. We feel what our mother feels. If we are fortunate to have a loving mother, (and father), we are set for life.

The most confusing thing to a baby's brain is indifference. Researchers say that the mother who hates her baby sends the clear signal the baby's brain needs to grow and differentiate.

The hated child will have problems the loved child will not, but will be better off than the child treated with indifference.

We need good **Limbic Resonance** for many years, as our brains keep growing and changing through our teens, and limbic resonance helps direct the growth. When deprived of good limbic resonance people can get violent and aggressive. Could this be why Americans are becoming more violent—could the lack of a good limbic connection account for the some of the mass killings?

Our need for limbic resonance never stops. As we grow older, we remain an open system. Our limbic system retains the need for contact. Resonance continues to change us. Who we love has a lot to do with who we become. Our significant emotional relationships change our brains, our feelings, and perhaps at the edges, our dispositions.

The impact of limbic connection is clear in the elderly. When one member of an elderly loving couple dies, the other feels that part of them has died too. In a way, it has: they have become as connected with their partner's brain as their own. When it dies part of them has died. Grief is even more understandable in this light, as is the fact that the surviving partner often leaves life quickly.

What does all this mean for us as conscious people? If we go into emotional resonance, if our limbic system has reasons we know not, and if our emotional triggers fire before we are aware, what does that mean? We can choose to change as we become more aware.

Maybe we get angry inappropriately. Maybe we fall in love with the wrong people. What we can do is learn to become aware of our emotional triggers more quickly. With the help of others, sometimes counseling, we can gain in awareness so that our emotions are not making decisions that harm us and are not foreclosing on emotions that would benefit us.

Talk therapy has no value in itself. We can't talk our way to happiness. It is healthy relationships that help heal. **When counseling works it is because love is present.** *And; God is love!*

It doesn't matter what opinions and ideas you try to tell yourself or others. It is a loving relationship with empathic attunement and connection that helps bring healing. If you go into resonance with someone who can give you the emotional cues you may not have had in earlier stages in life, you can learn from the resonance. Good teachers, good therapists, good counselors, good friends and good lovers all offer a successful resonance, one that emanates the love of Christ. We are open systems throughout our lives. That's what makes life worth living.

May we love one another with empathetic attunement in 'tangible' ways so that Christ's love is felt by our spouse and His healing is imparted into each life! Then the world will come to know Him by our love!

Female Anatomy

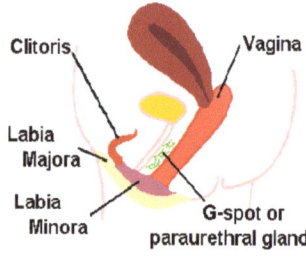

Female Ejaculation

Clitoris

Vagina

Labia Majora

Labia Minora

G-spot or paraurethral glands

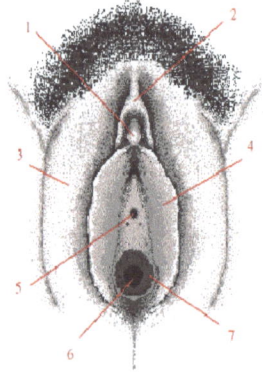

1 Clitoris

2 Clitoral Hood (prepuce)

3 Labia Majora (outer lips)

4 Labia Minora (inner lips)

5 Urethral opening

6 Vaginal opening

7 Hymen

Knowing anatomy is important for understanding how God has designed us. We are fearfully and wonderfully made for our existence and reproduction, as well as for our pleasure. We can worship God for His gift of our amazing anatomy and all the ways it functions.

Male Anatomy

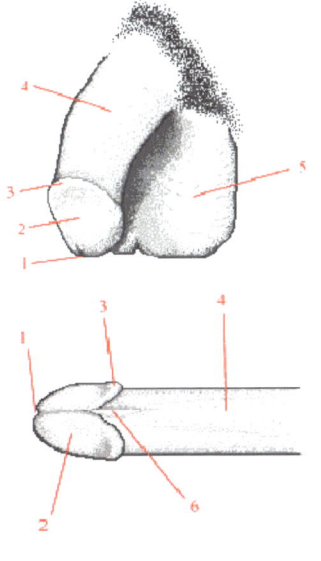

1 Urinary opening

2 Glans (head)

3 Corona (rim)

4 Shaft of penis

5 Scrotum

6 Frenulum

Knowing anatomy is important for understanding how God has designed us. We are fearfully and wonderfully made for our existence and reproduction, as well as for our pleasure. We can worship God for His gift of our amazing anatomy and all the ways it functions.

FEMALE ORGASM

Orgasm is a much more automatic response for men than for women. Orgasm isn't that easy, if you're a woman. Nearly all men can climax without difficulty, but women just aren't built that way. But many people don't realize this fact. Let's face it: books, films and magazines paint a different picture in which today's females are hot, raring to go and effortlessly orgasmic.

So, for women who are not all of these things — this type of media portrayal is, at best, unhelpful and, at worst, painful and damaging. Indeed, today's younger women tend to believe that there's something wrong with them — or even that they're frigid — if they can't climax to order. This is not the case. In fact, they're mostly absolutely normal.

Interestingly, however, only a generation ago many doctors used to believe that a high proportion of the female population simply couldn't climax at all. Why did they think this way? It was simply because most doctors had little or no training in sexual medicine.

Also, the majority of physicians were so embarrassed about sex themselves that they tried to avoid discussing it with their patients. Furthermore, since women don't need to climax in order to conceive, most doctors didn't rate the importance of the female orgasm very highly.

New attitude
Fortunately, doctors now have a different attitude. This is largely because they're now familiar with the results of sexual studies conducted by American researchers Kinsey, Masters and Johnson, Shere Hite and others.

In addition, the last 15 years have seen a number of sexual surveys conducted with large samples of people through newspapers and magazines. The results of these surveys have taken the lid off the sex life of the public.

Sex is not just for procreation. Sex and orgasm were created by God as one of the many ways we can worship Him. It is an amazing gift of intimacy and connection with Him, ourselves and our spouse.

It is now known that virtually any woman can climax — and indeed have multiple orgasms — **if the circumstances of her life are right**. And these circumstances usually include having a caring, understanding partner — who's knowledgeable about sex and who uses that knowledge to help her relax and to reach orgasm.

Orgasm is a much more automatic response for men than for women. It seems that even though there are plenty of deeply caring and decent men around, their ability to climax doesn't necessarily have to be linked to feelings of connection, love and romance.

Women of all ages, by contrast, tend to find that their sexual confidence and competence flower in a climate of appreciation and deep affection. To understand more about the female orgasm, let's go back to the start of a woman's sexual life.

The beginnings

A lot of young women are worried about their lack of ability to climax. But the fact is, unlike males, most females need to learn to reach orgasm. Research shows that most younger women do not manage to climax, until some considerable time after they have started sexual activity. Moreover, when they do orgasm for the very first time, they report doing it in a variety of ways. In one survey it was discovered that:

- 47 per cent climaxed for the first time through self stimulation
- 32 per cent through sexual intercourse
- 20 per cent through petting
- 1 per cent while sleeping.

In the same survey, it was found that the most common age of first orgasm was 18, but it could also be as late as the 40s!

The 20s and 30s

Even in their 20s and 30s, a lot of women have difficulty reaching that elusive orgasm. These days, most sex therapists believe that if you can't climax (or don't climax easily), it's a good idea to start by practicing on your own.

This may seem obvious, but many women, even today, feel inhibited about self exploration of their bodies and can't help feeling that it isn't something they should be doing. Ask God to show you what is right for you and do not engage in anything that is specifically prohibited in the Bible or that the Holy Spirit has convicted you as being a sin.

Self exploration and discovery can help you learn exactly which pressures and rhythms you need to come to orgasm. In particular you (or you and your spouse) may need to explore your body in order to find out precisely how to stimulate your clitoris and to find your G-spot.

Learning to explore and understand your own body should be an experience of valuing yourself and learning how to help your spouse bring you to orgasm. You can worship God for the wonder, beauty and joy of His gift of sex and orgasm.

Once you have learned what an orgasm is, and you are able to climax easily, you can then show your spouse exactly what you need for the sexual pleasure God intended. It may feel embarrassing at first, but it's important that you learn to communicate your feelings and how you like your body to be touched.

When you can't find the words, use caresses. But also, try to build up a vocabulary with your partner that's easy to use. A lot of couples find their sex lives fail simply because they don't have the right language. And saying: 'Could you rub my ...uh, ...um?' isn't specific enough to be helpful. You need to be clear and direct and both understand your bodies and how to use common vocabulary about your bodies and sexual experiences.

Some women, incidentally, find achieving orgasm much easier with the help of a vibrator. But for many females actually getting a marital sex aid that they can rely on isn't always easy. If this applies to you, there are several excellent Christian online mail order businesses that have been set up in the last decade or so. These marital sex aids can really help.

30 plus

By the time you are in your 30s, 40s or 50s: you should be able to reach orgasm quite easily — provided that you have a loving, understanding spouse. But do remember that most women find that their ability to climax varies according to what part of their menstrual cycle they're in, as well as their stage of menopause.

It's quite common for a woman to feel especially orgasmic half-way through her menstrual cycle. But some women feel particularly turned-on just before a period. Others notice that they don't really feel like sex at all during some times of the month. All of this is normal. If you're still not having any orgasms at all, or if you're still having difficulty 'getting there', it is definitely time to seek professional help.

Various types of orgasm

Thanks to Freud, the father of psychoanalysis, people used to believe that vaginal orgasms were what mature women had, while clitoral orgasms were what immature women had. Experts no longer believe this. And many of today's sex experts, as well as ordinary women, say that they really don't know the difference between a vaginal orgasm and a clitoral one. However, the majority of women need clitoral stimulation in order to climax.

A few women, on the other hand, believe they can climax through intercourse with no manual stimulation of the clitoris and claim that it's the vagina itself that sparks off the orgasm. Every woman is unique.

But many sex experts think that what's happening during intercourse is the clitoris is being stimulated by being pulled down or being rubbed by part of the man's torso. There's also the G-spot to consider. Some women experience a particularly intense orgasm when that part of their anatomy is stimulated (you can find the G-spot inside you, on the front vaginal wall). Many women who enjoy having their G-spots touched claim that they ejaculate during these intense orgasms.

So, there may be a case for saying that there's a G-spot orgasm — as well as possibly a vaginal one and one that originates in the clitoris.

It really doesn't matter whether or not there are different types of orgasms. The important thing is that you should be having good, reliable orgasms in your sex life. It is God's gift and desire for you by His amazing design.

Simultaneous orgasm

A lot of women complain that they can't reach simultaneous orgasm with their partners. But in fact, simultaneous orgasm is quite uncommon. Surveys done by the Medical Information Service and others have found that most women rarely climax at exactly the same time as their partners.

However, it's certainly nice when this happens. And it can be achieved — if the man has good control of his own orgasm and if he's skilled at using his fingers or a vibrator during intercourse — to bring the woman to a climax just at the same moment as he comes to orgasm. Or she may choose to use her own fingers or a vibrator to stimulate herself, so that they climax together.

Multiple orgasms

Until quite recent years, doctors believed that only a tiny minority of women could have multiple orgasms. But research by the Medical Information Service and others has shown that in fact, the majority of females can have a series of climaxes, one after the other if, that is, they're happy and relaxed in the relationship and if the partner is willing to stimulate them to come to orgasm again and again. The ability to have multiple orgasms increases with age. It's unusual at the age of 20, but many women in their 40s, 50s and 60s can do it.

Orgasms in mid-life

Again, a woman's ability to climax tends to improve with age. We know that some women get well into mid-life before they manage to have an orgasm. But the important thing is that you should never regard it as 'too late'. Time and again we have heard of women who have learned to orgasm when they were in their 40s, 50s — and even later.

In February 2009, at the Royal Society of Medicine, Danish psychosexual therapist Pia Struck presented the results of a study she had made of 500 women.

These women all had long histories of difficulties with orgasm and 25 per cent of them had never climaxed. Their ages ranged from 18 to 88. They were helped through the Betty Dodson method and were treated by use of group therapy, where they were encouraged to think more positively about their sexuality and learn acceptance of their genitals through touch. They also embarked on practical sex-therapy by using clitoral vibrators. Of these women: 465 (93 per cent) had an orgasm. And it was reported that the post-menopausal women among them were just as able to achieve orgasm as the younger participants in the study. So, clearly, you are never too old to become orgasmic.

There can of course be other problems in midlife, around the time of the menopause. Most of these difficulties occur because of all the hormonal changes going on in the body. And it's extremely common for women to 'go off' sex temporarily simply because it becomes too dry and uncomfortable. Fortunately, there are all sorts of ways to remedy this nowadays. There are good over-the-counter lubricants, such as Wet, Silk, Astroglide, Senselle and K-Y Jelly. These are all suitable, by the way, for any age of woman. Always check with your healthcare professional before trying any lubricants.

In mid-life, there's also the option of going on Hormone replacement therapy (HRT). But this is something that any woman should think about very carefully indeed. Until recently, it was widely believed that HRT commonly helped a woman to feel much better generally, and to feel sexier in particular. However, the picture has now changed significantly.

Extensive research into HRT now suggests that though it's still effective for ridding a woman of unpleasant menopausal symptoms — such as hot flushes and sweating attacks — it's not safe to use long term. So, it should definitely not be viewed as a magical youth elixir that you start taking at the menopause and continue using till you're an elderly lady. Many women find that health supplements, such as soya and red clover, also alleviate menopausal symptoms and actually help them to feel younger and fitter too. It must be stressed that the use of supplements is in its infancy, and you need to consult a healthcare provider before putting yourself on them.

If you are no longer able to engage in sexual intercourse with your partner, due to age, disabilities, or other issues, your relationship can still be a ten. Fulfilling relationship intimacy is still possible without intercourse.

How can men help?

- Remember that love, romance, cuddling and a good atmosphere turn women on in the early stages of a sex session — just as much as your caresses do.
- Do tell her often and sincerely that she's marvelous, sexy and beautiful. Be aware that many women feel insecure about the appearance of their bodies, especially if they are overweight or have a low self-esteem.
- Remember that most women need stimulation of the clitoris. It's just as important to women as the penis is to a man.
- Take your time. Don't rush. Ask her what she wants and likes. When she is properly aroused she will 'beg' for your penis to enter her vagina.
- Caress her breasts — a few women learn to climax through breast fondling alone.
- Give her oral sex if you both agree it is an allowable in your marriage. Most women adore this and some claim that they cannot come to orgasm unless a man orally or manually stimulates their clitoris.
- Don't be too proud to ask her to show you what she wants.
- Don't hesitate to use a vibrator, if she likes the idea and you both agree it is okay in your marriage.
- Have sex sessions, where you encourage her to take the initiative and make the agenda.
- If you lose control and orgasm before her, do try to summon some energy to kiss and stimulate her, so that she can climax too.

Summing up

Having an orgasm is wonderful. You're entitled to it. It is a gift created by God. But it's not easy to do if you're uptight, tired, stressed or unhappy in your relationship. If you have difficulty, seek help from a doctor, pastor or counselor. And remember relationship intimacy can still be satisfying and fulfilling without sex and orgasm.

FEMALE EJACULATION

The following assumes you have already an understanding of the G-spot. Women lactate, men ejaculate, or so the old saying goes. Turns out some women, maybe most women, actually do both. Reports of women experiencing a gush of fluid at orgasm go back many centuries, but it's only recently that (Western) science has taken these stories seriously.

Many still explain away the fluid some women eject from the urethra at climax as urine resulting from momentary loss of bladder control. While this *might* occur in a very small number of women, it does not explain the experience shared by some women: the fluid doesn't look like urine, doesn't smell like urine, and it has been proven in many chemical analyses that it is not urine. These women produce a small amount of clear fluid which has only trace amounts of uric acid; this indicates the fluid comes through the urethra, but **does not come from the bladder**. Chemically the fluid is very similar to the fluid from the male prostate.

Study has shown that the fluid comes from the "female prostate", more properly known as the paraurethralglands, and often referred to as the G-Spot. During gestation the male and female start with the same tissues, it's only after sex differentiation at about 40 days that the genitals begin to look different in the male and female fetus. The tissue which becomes the prostate in the male does not just disappear in the female, it becomes the paraurethral glands which surround the urethra. Based on postmortem dissections, we know that the amount of glandular tissue varies from woman to woman, and some women have no discernible glandular tissue in their G-spot.

In some women the paraurethral glands produce fluid when the woman is highly aroused. Because the paraurethral glands open into the urethra, the muscle contractions of orgasm force this fluid into the urethra, and out of the body, creating an ejaculation of sorts.

There are those who claim all women can "learn" how to ejaculate, but biology suggests otherwise; women who don't have any glandular tissue can't produce anything to ejaculate. Other woman may produce such a small amount of fluid that it's not noticed when mixed in with the other fluids that sex produces. Small amounts of fluid might not "squirt" out, but rather drip out after orgasm, much as semen does when a man has an almost-dry climax.

It's also possible that the fluid may leak out before orgasm; men have a sphincter (valve) "downstream" of the prostate that keeps fluid from leaking, but women have no such sphincter. It has also been speculated that in some women the fluid is sent "upstream" and into the bladder.

A few studies have shown some indication of female ejaculate in urine after orgasm, but it's not known if this is the result of a retrograde ejaculation or just the urine washing a small amount of fluid out of the urethra. In a recent study done by Dr. Santamaría Cabello[1], prostate-specific antigen (PSA) was found in the post orgasm urine samples of 75% of the women studied. The PSA could only come from the paraurethral glands, indicating apparent ejaculation. Most of these women did not report an ejaculation, suggesting the amount of fluid was either small, or the ejaculation went into the bladder. With only 24 participants the study is somewhat limited, but it does suggest that most women ejaculate at least a little bit.

Lack of understanding of this phenomenon has caused some women great anguish. Worried that she is urinating, or accused of such by her husband, a woman may find the only way to avoid ejaculating is to not orgasm at all. Finding out they are normal, and convincing their husbands they are not "peeing" can make a world of difference. Ironically, growing awareness of female ejaculation has created another problem; women (or their husbands) who worry that there is something wrong with them because they **don't** ejaculate. Some folks have become "female ejaculation evangelists" claiming that all women can, and those who don't are missing out on the best sex they can have.

A part of the zeal these folks exhibit may be based on a bad assumption about cause and effect. Some women who ejaculate say their ejaculatory orgasms are better than their non-ejaculatory ones, and some seem to think the ejaculation causes the orgasm to be better.

A more likely hypothesis is that only strong orgasms cause ejaculation in those women who have the tissue to do so. The idea that the best "dry orgasm" of a non-ejaculator is inferior to the "wet orgasms" of ejaculators is not supported scientifically. Additionally, some women say their dry and ejaculatory orgasms are very different, and some of these women say they feel unsatisfied without a "real" or dry orgasm at the end.

Bottom line: no woman should feel she is being cheated because she doesn't have ejaculations. Whether you do or don't experience female ejaculations, just enjoy your sexuality the way God has made you. Even if a woman has a small ejaculation, it can be messy. The amount of semen a man ejaculates can make an incredibly large mess; and since female ejaculate is thinner than male ejaculate it can spread even more, sometimes up to 2 cups. Being subject to gravity it can quickly soak through several layers of towels and leave a wet spot on the bed. Some couples resort to waterproof mattress covers, but this is probably more extreme than necessary; a single towel with a layer of plastic under it is sufficient.

Female Ejaculation

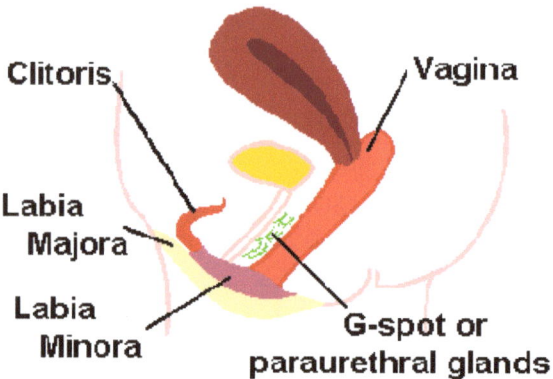

Knowing anatomy is important for understanding how God has designed us. We are fearfully and wonderfully made for our existence and reproduction, as well as for our pleasure. We can worship God for His gift of our amazing anatomy and all the ways it functions.

SEX POSITIONS

Creativity is critical for those who want to see an infusion of 'spice' into their marriage's sexual routine. Spice really is the excitement produced by variation. To that point, one of the common means of changing things up in the bedroom is in assuming different positions during sex. Certain positions vary the feel of penetration for both spouses. It also changes the visual perspective of what is going on and how our bodies experience one another.

The following are just a few of many variations of body positions during sex. Some would take very flexible spouses. Remember to agree together as a couple before you try any new sexual positions.

Side Positions:
Spoons- spouses lay side by side with their knees slightly bent. Man penetrates from behind as he "spoons" his wife.

Side-By-Side- husband and wife face each other and lay on their sides. T-square- woman lies on her back with her knees up and her legs open. Husband penetrates her at a perpendicular angle (he is on his side) their bodies form a "T".

Scissors- Woman is on her back, the man penetrates her from under one thigh. They interlock with their heads facing away from each other. (i.e. Take your index finger and your middle finger of both hands. Make a "V" or "peace sign with them...now interlock them. That's kind of how scissors works).

Missionary Positions:
Reverse Missionary- woman lays on top of her husband while he penetrates she controls the movement.

Spread Eagle- woman lies completely down. She is face down. Man lies on top of her and enters from the rear.

Coital Alignment Technique (CAT)-The man enters initially from between the woman's legs which are apart and slightly bent, but then lifts himself further up the length of her body so that his thrusts make contact with her clitoris.

Basically, this is a rocking back and forth in sync sort of thing with the focus on the clitoris and the base of the penis rather than being all about penetration. Depending on their relative height, she may be laying eye level with his chest versus eye to eye. This technique is highly praised by many and often leads to orgasm for women.

Woman On Top Positions:
Woman On Top (WOT) - wife straddles her husband as he lies on his back. She controls the penetration.

Reverse WOT- woman is again on top and straddling her husband, however this time she is facing AWAY from him.

WOT Crouching position — Woman straddles her husband, but she squats over him instead of Kneels. She then moves up and down in the squatted position

Reverse Missionary- woman lays on top of her husband while he penetrates she controls the movement.

Lotus Position- man kneels or sits cross legged and woman sits on top of him with her legs wrapped around him.

Lapdance- woman straddles her husband as he sits in a chair. She faces him.

Kneel Positions:
Kneel Style: Wife is on all fours. The husband penetrates from behind while on his knees. Classic.

Kneel Style (modified): A variant of the Kneel Style position is to have the wife angle the upper part of her body downward. The husband can raise his hips above hers to experience maximum penetration. In this position, the testicles may brush against the clitoris during forward thrusts providing additional stimulation to dear wife...

Kneel Style Upright: The husband squats (rather than kneels) behind her and penetrates. He places his hands on her back or waist to remain upright and stable. Of course, wife is on all fours.

Standing Positions:

Standing (modified): Wife faces away from dear husband. He penetrates from behind. She may use a wall as a brace and a means to allow both to be maximally aggressive.

Standing Suspense: Wife wraps her arms around his neck and legs around his waist. The husband, standing, penetrates her. The position is made easier when a supporting object like a wall (esp. in a corner) behind the wife is used. She may also sit at the very edge of a table, sofa back, bathroom sink or some other elevated surface.

Leg Lift: Husband stands behind wife. Wife places one foot on the seat of a chair and one hand on the chair back. She reaches back and holds his hand while he penetrates from behind. Husband uses his free hand to provide further stimulation.

Laid Back: Wife lies on the edge of the bed with her buttocks at the very edge and her feet on (toward) the floor. Husband stands between her legs and penetrates. A variation of this would be the wife placing her legs around his waist.

Pile Driver: The wife is on her back and lifts her hips and legs as high in the air as she can. The husband, standing, penetrates her vaginally while holding on to her legs to support her. This position requires downward thrusting and typically cannot be maintained very long by either partner.

Wheelbarrow: The wife rests her upper body on a padded chair. The husband, from behind, lifts her legs to his sides and penetrates her. Imagine holding a wheelbarrow! Standing (modified): Wife faces away from dear husband. He penetrates from behind. She may use a wall as a brace and a means to allow both to be maximally aggressive.

EROGENOUS ZONES

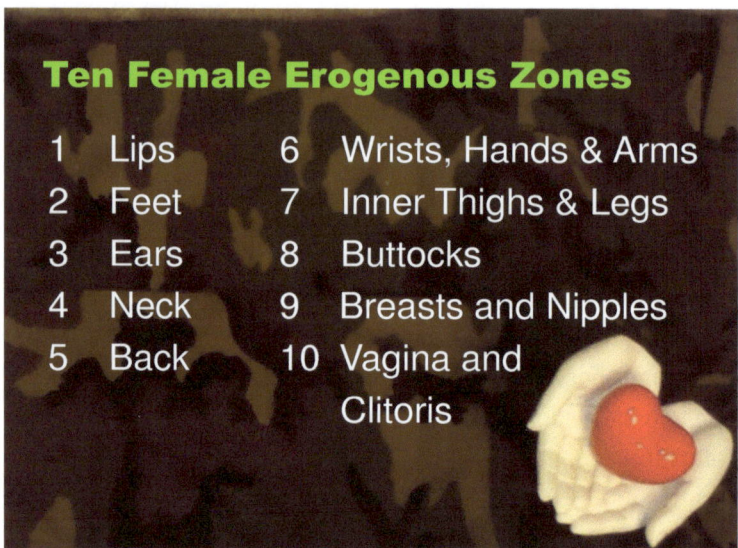

Ten Female Erogenous Zones

1	Lips	6	Wrists, Hands & Arms
2	Feet	7	Inner Thighs & Legs
3	Ears	8	Buttocks
4	Neck	9	Breasts and Nipples
5	Back	10	Vagina and Clitoris

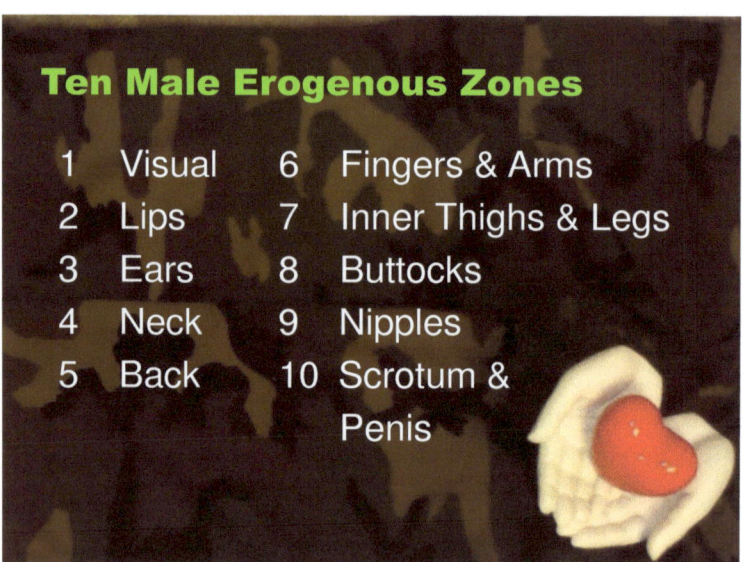

Ten Male Erogenous Zones

1	Visual	6	Fingers & Arms
2	Lips	7	Inner Thighs & Legs
3	Ears	8	Buttocks
4	Neck	9	Nipples
5	Back	10	Scrotum & Penis

HEALTH BENEFITS OF SEX

- Sex increases the levels of Oxytocin, a hormone associated with contentment.
- Sex decreases the stress hormones, thus improving the immune system.

The biologic benefits of sex are equal for both sexes. The health benefits of sex cannot be underestimated. Some of these benefits are:

1. Lower incident of illness
2. Relieve tension! The faster heartbeat, the increased blood flow and muscular tautness- relieving built up tension in the nervous system.
3. Improves self-esteem and provides a closer emotional attachment
4. Calm your cravings for junk food and sometimes for cigarettes. Sexual stimulation activates the production of a natural amphetamine that regulates your appetite.
5. Can work as Natural Pain Management. Endorphins can increase your tolerance to pain by as much as 70% during orgasm.
6. Helps you sleep better. Orgasms act as a natural tranquilizer, releasing the same endorphins that are released during exercise. That wonderful release of endorphins is very calming.
7. Burns calories. Enhances physical fitness levels.

Recognize the benefits of valuing sex the way it was created by God to be valued.   Sex is a gift that God gave men and women, and it is to be enjoyed fully in the monogamous relationship of marriage between a man and a woman. The Song of Solomon portrays a very detailed description of this passionate relationship between a man and women in love.

Be a Gutsy Sexual Man or a Sexual Super Woman. It is time for Christian men and women to promote a healthy perspective of sex. This issue too often goes unspoken and hidden. Let's take the "fig leaves" off in our marriages. Sex is a gift from God, and it is something to be enjoyed.

Sex is a part of an abundant life. The more open women are about sexuality, the more able they are to enjoy their own married sex life.

In John 10:10 Jesus said: "I came that they may have and enjoy life, and have it in abundance (to the full, till it overflows)".

An integral part of a healthy and abundant married life is a 'Gutsy Sex' life. A good sex life will strengthen one's marriage and improve your health. As married women, we should encourage one another to work through our difficulties and stereotypes, and help equip each other toward 'GUTSY SEX' and better health.

LOVE COUPON EXAMPLES

Consider creating your own Love Coupons to help increase your connection with your spouse and to assist you in growing your intimacy with one another.

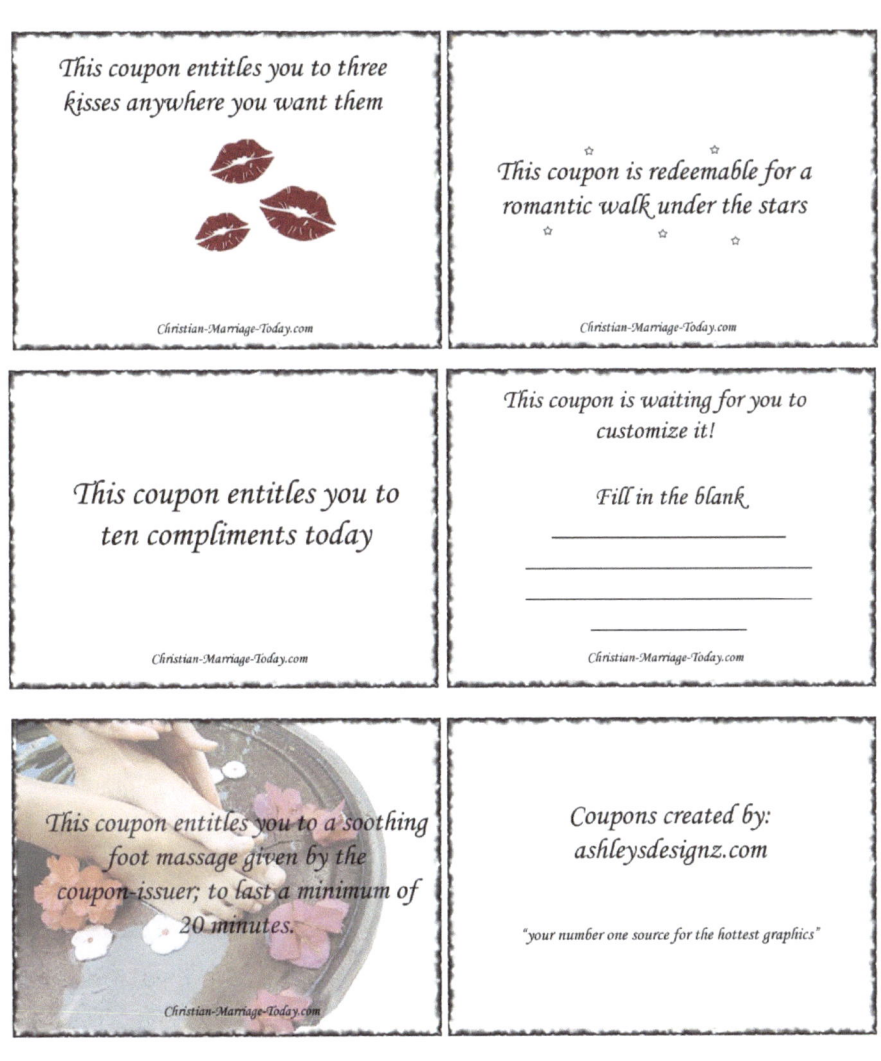

This coupon entitles you to three kisses anywhere you want them

Christian-Marriage-Today.com

This coupon is redeemable for a romantic walk under the stars

Christian-Marriage-Today.com

This coupon entitles you to ten compliments today

Christian-Marriage-Today.com

This coupon is waiting for you to customize it!

Fill in the blank

_____
_____
_____
_____

Christian-Marriage-Today.com

This coupon entitles you to a soothing foot massage given by the coupon-issuer; to last a minimum of 20 minutes.

Christian-Marriage-Today.com

Coupons created by:
ashleysdesignz.com

"your number one source for the hottest graphics"

RESOURCES

If you want to learn more about how to experience and extend love and enjoy 'Gutsy Sex', consider these resources. They can help you fulfill Mark 12:30-31. They will help deepen your intimacy with your spouse. Consider viewing, reading and discussing these resources together as a married couple. If you want more help seek someone trained to assist you with relationship problems. Most licensed counselors and pastors can help you with relationship and sexual issues.

Books

Pure Desire *by Ted Roberts*
        Spiritual Faith Focus **(HEART)**
Journey to the Other Side of Life *by Kevin Lane Turner*
        Emotional Feeling Focus **(SOUL)**
Discovering the Mind of A Woman *by Ken Nair*
        Mental Thought Focus **(MIND)**
Intended for Pleasure *by Ed Wheat, M.D. and Gaye Wheat*
        Physical Action Focus **(STRENGTH)**

Websites

There are some good online resources if you are interested in finding more information to help you experience 'Gutsy Sex'. Below are two that may be helpful.

www.themarriagebed.com
www.gamesforloving.com

This "Gutsy Sex' Guide includes information from various resources, trainings and seminars written and/or attended by the LifeCare Counseling Ministry Team since 1981 including knowledge acquired from: the National Christian Counselors Association; Roger Martin, Center for Research, University of Kansas; A General Theory of Love, by Thomas Lewis, Fari Amini; Richard Lannon; Daniela Roher, PhD, LPC.; Paul Ekman, PhD and numerous other books and online public domain resources.

AUTHOR

Pastor Debbie Horton, LCPC, has been involved in Christian counseling ministry since 1978. Her college years and personal therapy taught her the value of coupling clinical knowledge with Biblical principles. She is trained in Christian Counseling Psychology, Gestalt Therapy, Integrated Marriage and Family Therapy, Temperament Therapy, Domestic Violence Treatment, Trauma and Abuse Recovery Therapy and Paramedic and Nursing patient care. Her wisdom, warmth, humor and prophetic insight help create a compassionate and safe relationship where you will feel free to explore, grow and improve your life journey, whether in person or through her writings. With nurture and understanding, she works with each individual to help them build on their strengths and attain the personal growth they are committed to accomplishing. As a NCCA Licensed Clinical Pastoral Counselor she holds a master's degree in Christian Counseling Psychology and is a licensed ordained minister with Grace International. She is a seasoned Christian Therapist, Teacher and Writer.

LifeCare Publishing
Roseburg, Oregon
www.lifecarecounselors.com

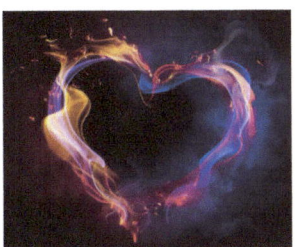

9 7 8 1 4 7 8 2 9 3 8 2 8